Home Workout

The Home Workout Plan On How To Get Fit For Life

Elle Petersen

2

Table of Contents

Introduction

I want to thank you and congratulate you for downloading the book, *"Home Workout For Beginners: The Home Workout Plan on How to Get Fit for Life"*.

This book contains a plan, recommendations and exercises on how to get fit by working out at home.

Going to the gym can be difficult, either we have so many excuses of not going to the gym for a workout or we have no access to the gym. Many gyms are also just too loaded with people, that it is actually hard to work out once you get there. You don't want to waste your money and extra time on going to a gym like that. Exercising at home is actually easier than you might think and works just as well. This book will help you staying fit and toned while staying at home.

The exercises this book contains require no equipment at all. You can easily do them at home. I will present additional tools for those who might be interested. The exercises are highly effective and will help you in toning down your body, building muscles and much more. Some of the exercises are also given with a warning to prevent you from any injuries and wrong doing. The workouts are absolutely safe! Follow the steps properly and see the difference on your body yourself. Not only will you look good, you will also feel more relaxed and have more energy, after having tried this simple program on working out.

You will find, in this book, a total body workout routine which includes core exercises, arms exercises, upper back and lower back exercises and a lot more. There is definitely something for everyone here.

Thank you again for downloading this book, I hope you enjoy it and I wish you good luck!

Elle Petersen

Chapter 1: Why and how is exercise important?

"Use it or lose it", have you heard this expression before? It is so true! You need to use your body or else you will lose it. Using your body means exercising and if you don't, then your body becomes weak and flabby. Body organs like lungs and heart will be unable to function effectively and your joints will become so stiff that they would get injured easily. Inactivity risks your health like smoking does!

1. Controls Weight

Exercise is one of the keys to controlling your weight as it burns calories. It not only helps in losing weight, but it also helps in maintaining the weight loss. You lose weight when you burn more calories than the amount you have taken in. Calories could be burnt by working out daily at home or at the gym. If you find it difficult to take the time for exercise, then try doing things like household chores or taking stairs instead of an elevator.

2. Helps Prevent Diseases

Did you know that our bodies crave for exercise? -they were meant to move. Exercising regularly is important for good health and physical fitness. It reduces the risk of cancer, diabetes, high blood pressure, heart disease and other diseases. Exercise can delay the process of aging and can make you look young and healthy.

3. Enhances Flexibility

Stretching exercises are important as they improve your postures. Stretching makes your body limber i.e. twisting, bending and moving become easier. If you improve your flexibility by exercising, there are fewer chances that you injure yourself. It also ameliorates your coordination and balance. Those people, who have tense, stiff areas, like the neck or upper back, they can loosen their muscles by performing stretching exercises, and this will make them feel relaxed.

4. Improves Stamina

When you are exercising, your body is utilizing the energy in order to keep you going. Aerobic exercise calls for rhythmic and continuous physical motion, like bicycling and walking. It helps in improving your stamina and trains your body in utilizing less energy when working out and makes it more efficient.

5. Strengthens and Tones

Exercising makes your bones and muscles strong. It tones your body and enhances your physical appearance. It makes you feel and look better.

6. Improves the Quality of Life

By exercising regularly, you begin to feel better and more confident. Exercising makes you sleep better and reduces stress. If you make a habit of exercising, the process of aging will be easier for you. You will feel at good health for a longer time.

How often should you exercise?

Exercising daily is a healthy habit, it keeps you fit. A "stop start" routine won't benefit at all. Consistency is required once you begin to workout. On days when you don't feel like exercising then do simple stretches or climb the stairs of your house, four to five times a day.

Our bodies release "endorphins" when we exercise regularly and this helps in enhancing our moods. When you don't exercise for days or weeks, you feel low and there is a decrease in your energy level.

When you regularly exercise it makes you feel revived; mentally and physically. With a consistent exercise routine, the muscles develop gradually and mentally you will feel less stressful and more relaxed.

CAUTION

- Avoid doing intense exercises daily. This is harmful to your body and can result in fitness-level plateaus, loss of lean tissue and muscle strains.
- Beginners should always start slowly. Do not rush on things. There are no shortcuts in life.
- According to World Health Organization (WHO) an individual should exercise 30 minutes a day or walk for an hour. This is not to lose weight but a daily routine every person should follow, this is the requirement of our body.
- Keep your bodies working!

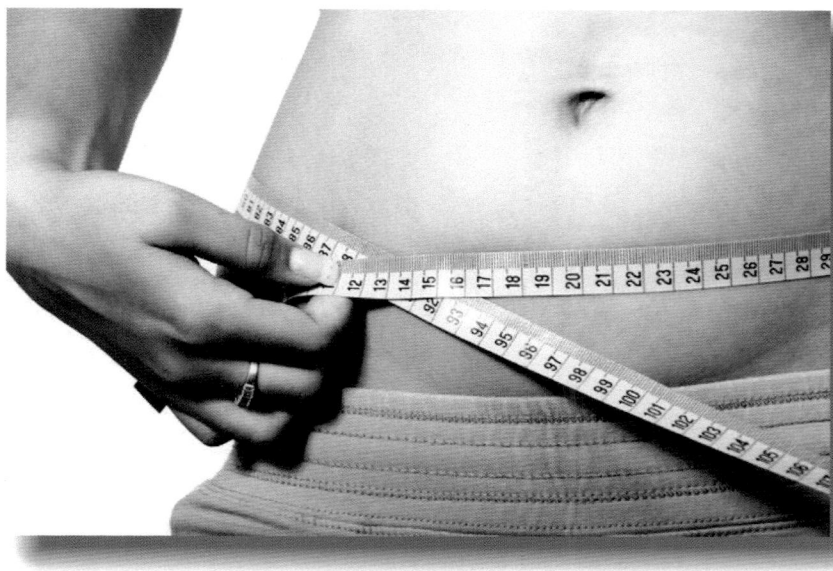

Chapter 2: The vital role of healthy eating

'The food you eat can be either the safest and most powerful form of medicine or the slowest form of poison." – Ann Wigmore

Indeed, our overall health and wellbeing is largely determined by the particular types of food that we usually consume in our day to day lives. Our diet plays a huge part in allowing us to maintain a healthy immune system to help fight diseases and infection and also in providing us with the strength and energy needed for us to function at our optimum daily.

A lot of individuals, however, often get intimidated by the idea of dieting since what mostly comes into mind is a kind of strict diet which exceedingly deprives them of the types of food they love to eat. But in contrast to this fairly common notion, it is very important to be aware of the fact that the best diet for a healthier body is not really about eating less but rather about eating what is right.

To be able to maintain optimum nutrition, it is very necessary for us to have a balanced diet - that is, obtaining the right types and the right proportions of food that will help supply the best nutritional value and energy which are vital for maintaining the cells, tissues, and organs of the body, which in turn, will support optimum growth, development and function.

Maintaining a Well Balanced Diet

Individuals have varying health needs and as such, it is advised to seek the advice of a certified health care professional, dietician, or nutritionist regarding what specific types of food will suit your needs most. But generally, a healthy and well balanced diet is composed of the following major food groups:

a) Fruits and Vegetables

Fruits and veggies are very important components of our diet since they are among the best sources of the essential vitamins and minerals vital to the optimum functioning of the body. Generally, it is advised to consume at least five portions daily, with each portion coming from a different fruit and vegetable to ensure that you obtain a variety of vitamins, minerals and other nutrients.

b) Protein

Protein is another essential food group which plays a major role in the building, repair, and maintenance of body tissues. Protein may come either from vegetable or animal sources. Vegetable sources include whole grains, buts and beans while the best animal sources include fish and poultry.

Red meat is also a source of protein. However, this particular protein source is known to contain high levels of saturated fat which could bring unpleasant effects to the body. As such, only the leanest cuts must be chosen in moderate portion sizes and must be made only an occasional component of your diet.

c) Dairy

Dairy is a very rich source of calcium, which is very vital not just in promoting and maintaining strong bones and teeth but also in helping regulate muscle contraction, including the beating of the heart. Basic dairy foods include milk, cheese and yoghurt. For individuals who are lactose intolerant, other calcium sources are dark green leafy vegetables, including spinach and broccoli, almonds, calcium-fortified soya milk, and certain types of fish.

d) Carbohydrates

Being the body's main source of energy, carbohydrates should be a part of each meal in general. However, it is important to keep in mind that there are good and bad carbohydrates out there. Bad carbs are those which lack nutrients needed by body and include several processed foods such as pastries, candies, cookies and sodas.

Good carbs, on the other hand, are those which are nutrient-filled and provide lots of benefits to the body. These include whole grains, legumes, and fruits and vegetables. Whole grain products are considered to be the best type of carbohydrates since they are known to contain fiber which is beneficial in having a healthy digestive system. They also contain several vitamins and minerals, protein, and even a rich content of antioxidants which could help prevent certain diseases such as cancer, diabetes and heart disease.

e) Fats

Unlike the common notion that fats should be totally avoided, it is very important to keep in mind that fats are also an essential part of any healthy diet. They play an important role in transporting fat-soluble vitamins, such as vitamins A, D, E and K, all throughout the body. They also help provide your body with energy, provide insulation in order to regulate your body temperature, and supply the body with essential fatty acids which play an important role in blood clotting, inflammation management, and even brain development.

As such, fats must not be entirely eliminated from our diet. We just have to be able to choose the 'good' fats from the 'bad' ones. Some of the healthiest fat choices are:

> *Monounsaturated Fats* – These are fats which are beneficial for the heart and are considered to be good sources of the antioxidant vitamin E. Some sources of this kind of fat are olives, sesame seeds, hazelnuts, pumpkin seeds, avocados, cashews, almonds, olive oils, peanut oils, and canola oils.

> *Polyunsaturated Fats* – These are fats which help lower the triglyceride levels and blood cholesterol levels of the body. They can be found in walnuts, flaxseed, and omega-3 fatty acids in certain fatty fish, such as salmon.

Keeping it in moderation and going natural are the key principles when it comes to maintaining a diet which is essential for a fit and healthy body. This denotes that we must consume only as much as what is truly needed by our body and must learn to limit our intake of sugary, salty and processed foods, although occasional treats and indulgences are considered alright.

Our body has a number of complex functions and to ensure that these essential functions are supported to always be at their optimum, we are required to make an effort to be mindful about what we feed our body with and to always be reminded of our aim to balance what is truly needed to sustain a fit and healthy body.

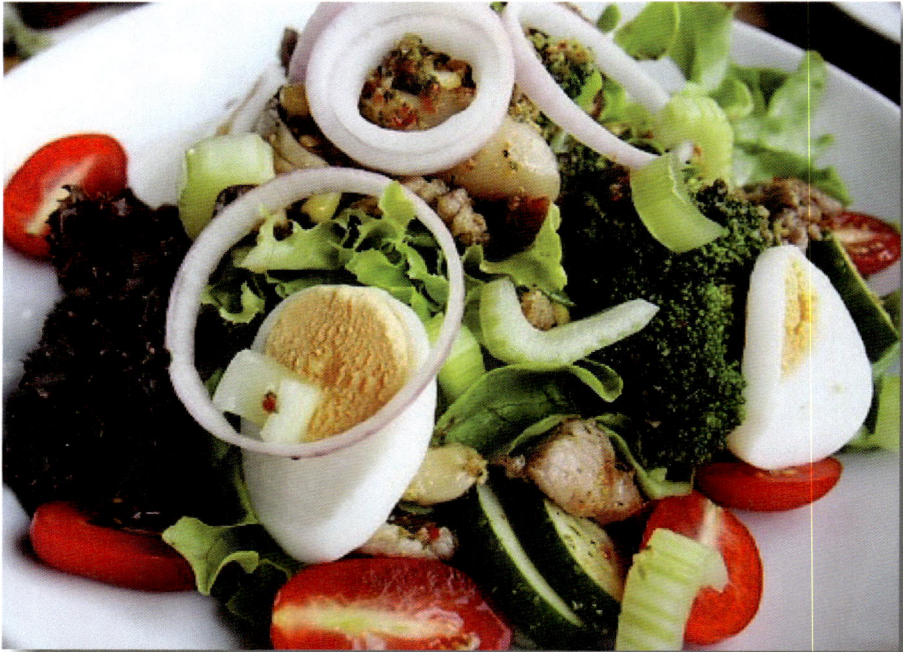

Chapter 3: Make a plan

Once you have decided to workout at home, you need to make a proper plan. This plan will include your daily diet and the number of minutes or hours you work out. Once you have a plan, you will feel even more motivated. Note down whatever you eat and the things you do over the day. After a week, assess what your calorie intake etc. is. This will help you to check and spot where things go wrong.

5 Elements of Fitness

You can do all of the following at home:

- A warm-up.
- A cardiovascular/aerobic workout.
- Strength-building exercises.
- Flexibility moves.
- A cool down

The warm-up can be a simple walk on a treadmill or outside, or riding a bike in a slow pace. If you are doing a cardiovascular workout then, walk/ pedal faster, jump rope or do step aerobics by watching a video – anything that you enjoy doing increases your heart rate.

The strength building exercises could be as simple like abdominal crunches, push-ups, and squats. If weight bars, tubing or bands or small dumbbells are available at home, you can work out with them. If these are not available but you wish to do such a workout then take plastic bottles and fill them with water, they will work like small dumbbells.

To increase your flexibility, you could do yoga poses or floor stretching. Then comes the cool down which should be similar to your warm up. A cool down is basically to bring down your heart rate at a resting state.

* Doing squats (without weights or with weights) works the calves, hamstrings, quadriceps, and gluteus.

*Push-ups involve the triceps, biceps, deltoids, pectorals -- even the upper back and the abdominals.

Getting started

You have decided to start exercising. Great! You have taken the first step towards a better and improved mind and body.

Exercise is known to be a magic pill. It can cure heart diseases, prevent and helps in recovering from cancer, helps people who have arthritis and helps in preventing and reversing depression.

Any physical activity is an exercise as it allows your body to move and engages your mind. There is absolutely no need for a heavy gym workout. There are numerous exercise options you can do at home, such as:

- Dancing
- Biking
- Gardening
- Doing household chores
- Walking

Do what you enjoy the most!

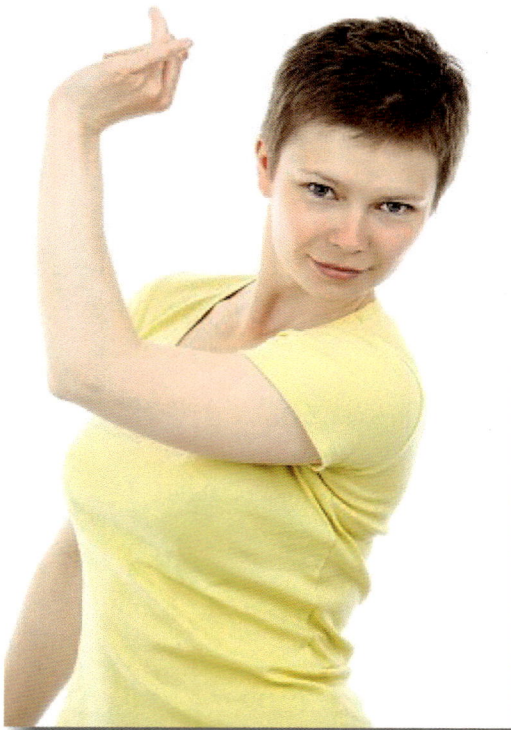

If you are a beginner, then you should do 30 minutes of cardiovascular workout three times every week, and about 20-30 minutes of a strength workout, at least three times in a week. Your strength workouts should involve your upper and lower body, your back, and your abdominal muscles.

No matter what type of workout you are doing, be sure to start slow and then gradually you could increase the intensity and time of a workout. If you start with high-intensity workout, they can cause cramps and other muscle problems to occur. Always listen to your body. Don't exhaust yourself.

The important thing to remember is that when you are working on a muscle, you should feel it. When working on your abs, you should feel it in your abs and not in your neck.

Working out at home

Exercising at home has many advantages, sometimes followed by obstacles. Obstacles include: distractions from the kids, the phone, the internet, the refrigerator and the dog etc. In order to avoid these distractions, experts advise you to exercise early in the morning.

Chapter 4: Easy and simple home workouts

Don't forget to warm up before you start exercising and once you are done don't forget to cool down.

Note: warming up and cooling down can just be a short walk or a jog.

The workouts given below are quick and simple and can be done at home. They can either be performed once in a day or you can even do them twice or thrice in a single day. They are more or less designed to fit a busy lifestyle. Something is better than nothing at all, so a little exercise is better than not doing it at all. These exercises will assist in muscle building, fat loss and toning.

Note: if you are not used to exercising them, please don't do too much at one time, start slowly and gradually.

Some easy and effective exercises that can be performed at home are:

- Ab crunches
- Press ups

- Knee press ups
- Triceps' dips
- Knee raises
- Leg raises
- Pull-ups
- Star jumps

Keep changing your workouts so you don't get bored. Enjoy every exercise you do, the more you enjoy it, the more effective it will be for you. Concentrate on what you do!

- **Ab crunches**

The abdominal crunch is one of the best exercises for strengthening the abdominals. If you have no idea on what this exercise (or any of the following) looks like, simply google it for images and you'll get a lot of examples.

- **Abdominal crunch:**

First of all, lie down on your back (keep the back flattened). Knees should be bent at a 90-degree angle and feet should be flat on the floor. Then place the hands behind your head. (Starting position which is also used for abdominal crunch twist)

Keep your head in line with the body and avoid pushing your head forward. Now you will have to slowly and steadily lift up the shoulders and head in order to perform this crunch. Instantly you will feel your abdominals are being worked out, and then slowly start lowering yourself. Do it in 4 steps and repeat it 20 times.

- **Abdominal crunch twist**:

The twisting motion in these crunches will target your oblique and the muscles at the side of abdominal.

Get in the same position like you do for a normal crunch (mentioned above). Once you have taken the position, place your left fingers on the left side of your head (temple area), then slowly lift your shoulders and your head up and twist while pointing your left elbow to your right knee and then slowly lower down. On the same side repeat for at least 10 times and then switch sides.

- **Bicycle crunch**

Take the same position like you do for a normal crunch.

Twist your body. Move your left elbow towards your right knee, extend and then straighten the other leg while keeping it a few inches off the ground.

You will feel your oblique and abdominals being worked out as you do this exercise. If you don't feel it then that means you are not doing it right. Repeat this with the other side as well.

• **Press ups/Knee press ups (chest exercise)**

The press up is an effective and a simple exercise that only requires your own body weight. It's excellent for developing and working your shoulders, arms and chest. It is also used for building muscles and for toning up the body.

Place knuckles or palms on the ground and hand to be placed wider than the width of the shoulder.

Legs and body should be kept straight. Lower yourself slowly till your chest is almost touching the floor.

Push your body back up slowly, until the arms are completely or nearly straight. If you bend your arms slightly it will give more tension on your muscles.

• **Knee press ups**

Get down on your knees and palms. Your knees should be bent at about a 90 degrees angle. Support the weight of your lower body, your arms should be straight and thighs to be vertical.

Lower your body slowly till your chest is almost touching the floor, then push your body back up again.

For increasing the body weight resistance, lean forward on the arms.

This is great for beginners as it requires less of your body weight.

- **Triceps' dips (arm exercise)**

This exercise can also easily be performed at home, all you require is a bench, bed or chair to do this exercise.

Triceps dip/dip is an exercise which develops and works multiple muscles such as shoulders, triceps, and chest.

If you are doing it with a bench;

Hands should be behind your body (shoulder width apart) and use your knuckles to hold onto the bench. Keep you face straight and look forward, your legs should be straight in front of you, together.

Arms should be slightly bent with straight legs. Now lower your body slowly and bend your elbows at a 90-degree angle. Your upper arms should be almost parallel to the ground.

Control your body and slowly return to the start position.

- **Leg raises and knee raises (abdominal exercise)**

Knee and leg raises are effective for training your abdominals, especially the hip flexor and the lower abdominal. The best thing about this exercise is that it can be performed at home as well as on a flat surface.

- Leg raises – raising your legs fully
- Knee raises – raising your knees only

Strong abdominals will help you in doing your daily activities. Your abs are the core muscles and are extremely important for basic physical movements, such as walking.

- **Leg Raises**

Perform this exercise on the floor or on a towel or on an exercise mat.

Lie down, keeping your back on an exercise mat or on the floor. Your hands should be under your butt (buttocks) and legs are supposed to be just a couple of inches off the floor.

Raise your legs slowly up bringing them in a vertical/almost vertical. Hold your legs there for a few seconds and then start lowering your legs till the legs are just a couple of inches off the floor. Repeat. Leg raises can also be performed on a bench. Keep your legs suspended off the benches' edge; this will increase the motion of this workout, giving you an added benefit.

- **Knee Raises**

"Leg raises" is a physically challenging exercise as it needs a good deal of abdominal strength. Some people might find it extremely difficult so they should start with knee raises.

Lie down with your back on an exercise mat or on the floor. Hands should be under your butt (buttocks), keep your legs a couple of inches off the floor. Bend the legs and then bring your knees up. Thighs should be in a vertical position and your knees should be bent at a 90 degrees angle. Straighten the legs. Repeat.

- **Pull ups (upper back exercise)**

"Pull ups" is a fantastic workout for working the "Latissimus Dorsi" (Lats) (this muscle gives you your back width). It also is great for the biceps. For performing this exercise you need to have a stronger upper body, however, with repetition and time your strength will get better.

Normally, pull ups require proper machines. But those who wish to perform this at home, can instead place a bench, table or a chair beneath them, and then they can push up with their legs.

Tip

You can use assistance as you are a beginner, with time you will gain strength to perform this exercise without any assistance.

- **Star Jump**

A star jump is an outstanding exercise. It tones your butt, your legs and turns your heart rate up.

Put your hands on your feet. Now all you have to do is to "explode" up like a star. It's very simple yet an intense exercise.

Squat down, then explode yourself up into a star and then get back down. Keep your hands to the toes, the head should be up and your back should be straight. Keep everything tight and nice. Explode up and then get back down to the start position. Repeat it at least 10 times.

Tips

If you want to do more, take a break for one minute. Repeat it. Take a break, and then repeat again. Do it in three sets by taking one minute break after every ten.

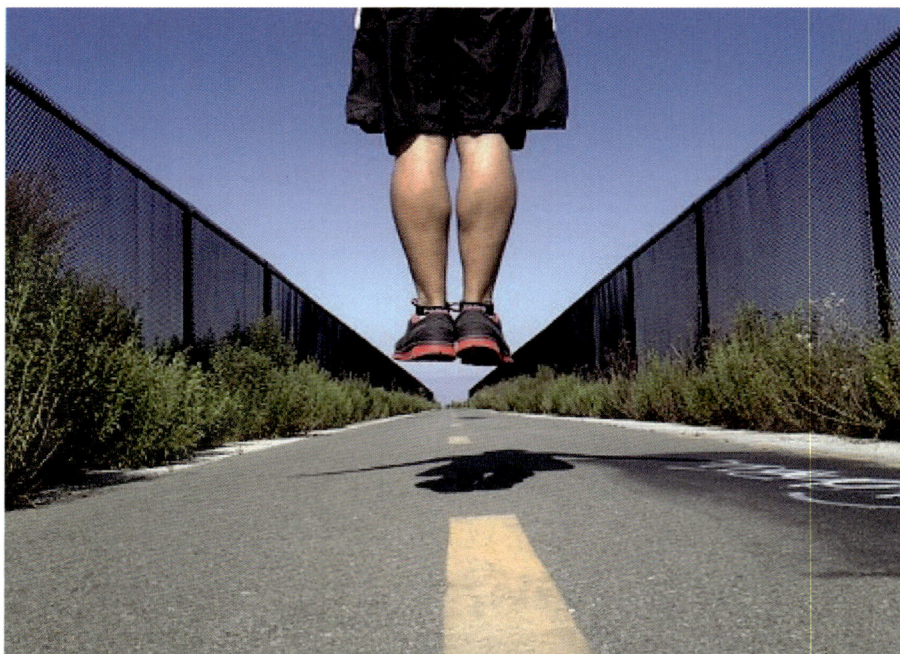

- **Rocket jumps**

Stand with your feet wide apart, bend your legs and keep your hands on your thighs. Jump! Your hands should be straight above the head while you jump. Repeat it.

To challenge yourself more, start with a "lower squat position" and hold in both your hands a water bottle or a weight, at the middle of your chest.

Tips

- Do two sets each of 15 repetitions.
- After doing this cardio exercise, jog or walk for 15 - 40 seconds.

- **One leg kickbacks (for lower back and buttocks)**

Put your body weight on your knees and hands. Your hands should be under the shoulders and knees under the hips. Keep your left leg bent at a 90 degrees angle and then raise your knee high (as much you possibly can) while squeezing your butt. Lower back to the start position and then with each leg repeat for 8 to 10 times.

Tips to remember:

- Keep your shoulders back and neck long.
- As you raise the leg, do not arch the back

- **Tap backs**

To start doing tap backs, step the left leg back and then swing both of your arms forward. Repeat in the same manner with the other leg. You need to look forward and your shoulders and hips should also be facing forward. As you step back, your front knee should not extend over your toes.

Do 2 sets each with 15 reps.

To make it more challenging, switch your legs by a jump. Always keep the knees soft while landing. At all times, the back heel will be off the ground.

- **Jumping Jacks**

Jumping jack is known to be a classic exercise which helps work out and stimulate almost every muscle in the body. It is known to increase heart rate and in turn, significantly help enhance blood flow to the different muscle groups.

To perform jumping jacks, simply stand straight with your feet together and your hands placed on your side. Then, in a single motion, jump your feet out to your sides and raise both your arms above your head. Reverse this motion by jumping back to the original position.

Chapter 5: Simple beginner body weight circuit

You don't need to go to a gym to lose those extra pounds and to look fit. Neither do you require any equipment. Do this simple beginner body weight circuit and you will see a difference.

How to do it: Do this workout as a circuit and complete, for each exercise, the given number of repetitions, without resting. You can rest for 2 minutes once you have completed one set of each exercise. Then repeat one to two more times, the entire circuit.

The exercise routine includes:

- 20 bodyweight squats
- 20 walking/side lunges
- 15 push ups
- 10 hip raise
- 15-30second plank
- 8-12 Floor Y-T-I Raises
- 10 dumbbell rows (use a gallon milk jug instead)

Exercise No. 1: Bodyweight Squat
Spread your feet apart a little wider than the width of your shoulder and stand as tall as it's possible for you. At the

shoulder level, straighten your arms in front of your body and hold them together making them parallel to the floor. For the entire movement, keep your body straight, with your lower back very slightly arched. Then brace your abs and lower the body as much as you can by pushing back the hips and by bending the knees. Pause for a few second and then push yourself back to start position. This is one repetition. Repeat it 15-20 times.

Exercise No. 2: Lunges

This is one of the best exercises to do for your glutes and thighs.

Stand straight, keeping your feet together, shoulders back and head up. Hands should be placed on the hips (if holding kettle bells or dumbbells keep your hands on your sides). Face forward and choose a place in order to keep your eyes focused while performing the exercise.

Now, take a lunge, with your first leg, forward (big lunge). Bend the forward leg at a 90-degree angle, while keeping your thigh parallel to the ground. Bend the back leg also at a 90-degree angle, with you back knee almost touching the ground. Keep your body as still and controlled as it's possible.

With your front leg, push yourself back up while pushing off with your front heel till you stand straight with feet together. Repeat this with the other leg as well.

Walking lunge: Do a normal lunge. Keep your feet together and lunge forward with your other leg again, so that you continue walking in a forward motion.

Side lunge: lunge out to the side while keeping your entire body weight on the heel of your lunging legs. Keep the other leg straight and by using the lunging leg heel and push your body back up.

*It's very important to do lunge in a proper way, to avoid strain on your joints.

**If you are unable to do the lunges or the body weight squats properly yet, then it's absolutely fine to place your hand on a support for balancing.

For body weight squats, think as if you are sitting back in a chair. If you are able to sit in a chair, and then stand up immediately without leaning forward that means you are in balance.

For lunges, you should keep your eyes in front and your upper body should be completely vertical.

Exercise No. 3: Incline Push-up

Assume that you are in a push-up position, but instead of placing your hands on the floor, you need to place your hands on a raised surface—like a bench or a box, or you can use the steps of the stairs.

Keep your body straight so that it forms a straight line (from your head to your ankles). Then lower the body, keeping it stiff, unless your upper arms "dip" below the elbows. Pause for a few seconds and then quickly push yourself again to the start position. (The higher you place your hands, the more easy the exercise becomes—you could also lean against the wall if you want to.) If you find this incline push-up too easy, then you can do it the "old-fashioned" way i.e. keep your hands on the floor. Repeat it 12 to 15.

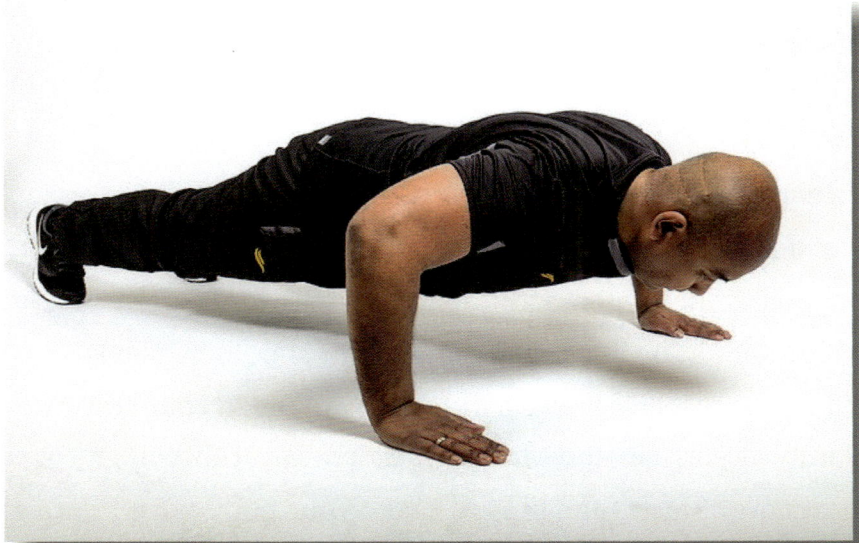

Exercise No. 4: Hip Raise

Lie down with your knees bent and back on the floor and keep your feet flat onto the floor. Place your arms out, at a 45 degrees angle, to your sides, with your palms facing upwards. Now try making your tummy skinny (as much as it's possible) and then hold it there—this will give you a tight core—while keeping your breathing normal. This is your starting position. Keep your core tight as much as you can, squeeze your gluteus and then raise your hips. Make sure your body is forming a straight line from shoulders to knees. Pause for about 5 seconds—keeping your glutes squeezed tightly this entire time—then slowly lower your body back to the start position. Repeat it 10 times.

Exercise No. 5: Side Plank

Lie down on your right side, keeping your knees straight. Support your upper body on your right forearm and elbow, which should be in line with your right shoulder. The left hand should be placed on your left hip. Try to make your stomach as skinny as you can and then hold it that way, this will give you a tight core. Raise your hips to make your body form a straight line from your shoulders to your ankles. Keeping your core tight and hold your body in this position for about 15 to 30 seconds. Change side and repeat.

Modified Side Plank

If you find side plank difficult, hold for 5 seconds then rest for about five seconds, and repeat (make it a total of 15 seconds). Each time while doing this exercise; try to hold a bit longer, so that you are able to reach your thirty-second goal.

If you still find it hard to do, bend the knees at 90 degrees and as you do the exercise, let your lower legs rest on the floor.

Exercise No. 6: Floor Y-T-I Raises

This exercise is a combination of three moves. You will have to repeat each exercise 8-12 times, one after the other, do not rest.

Repeat 8-12 times Floor Y raise, followed by 8-12 reps of Floor T raise, followed by 8-12 reps of Floor I raise.

Floor Y Raise

Lie on the floor with your face down, arms resting on the floor. Your arms should be straight, at a 30-degree angle to your body, so that they form a "Y." Your palms should face each other so that thumbs of your hand point up.

Floor T Raise

This will be performed just like Y raise, only you have to move your arms. Keep your arms out to your side (perpendicular to the body) with your thumbs pointing up and then raise them as high as you easily can.

Floor I Raise

This time you will move your arms in such a position so that the body forms a straight line from fingertips to your feet. Make sure your palms face each other, with your thumbs pointing up. Then raise your arms as high as you easily can.

Exercise No. 7: Dumbbell rows

Use a milk jug instead of a dumbbell or any other heavy thing. Find yourself something which is challenging to lift about 10 to 12 times in a row. Do this workout two to three times a week. Never do it on consecutive days.

Chapter 6: Additional tools for your workout

In this section, I would like to present you with a couple of tools that have added great value to my own home workout plan. The following tools do not cost much to purchase and you will be able to use them for many years ahead.

Using a Fitness Ball

One exercise tool that is easy to buy and use in your daily workout at home, if you feel you want to add something more, is the fitness ball (sometimes referred to as a gym ball or body ball etc.). If you want to purchase one of these, do talk to the sales person in the shop to make sure you buy one of a good size for you.

The fitness ball was essentially designed for light exercises, with the aim of treating people with orthopedic problems. In fact, it is still being used within physical therapy programs everywhere. It is also often used for Yoga and in athletic training. So why is it good to use? Well, it improves your body stability, balance and it engages muscles that you might normally not use that often.

A very good and easy exercise is to just sit on it, and perhaps move around a bit when you feel comfortable to do so. This way, your back and abdominal muscles get active in trying to reach a good and correct sitting posture for your body. Repeat this often and you will notice how it gets much easier to do. A lot of people nowadays actually use this method at the office in front of the computer. They switch their normal chair for a fitness ball for a period of time, perhaps 30 minutes or so, before they switch back. If you know that you are sitting still a lot as well, this might be a good idea for you.

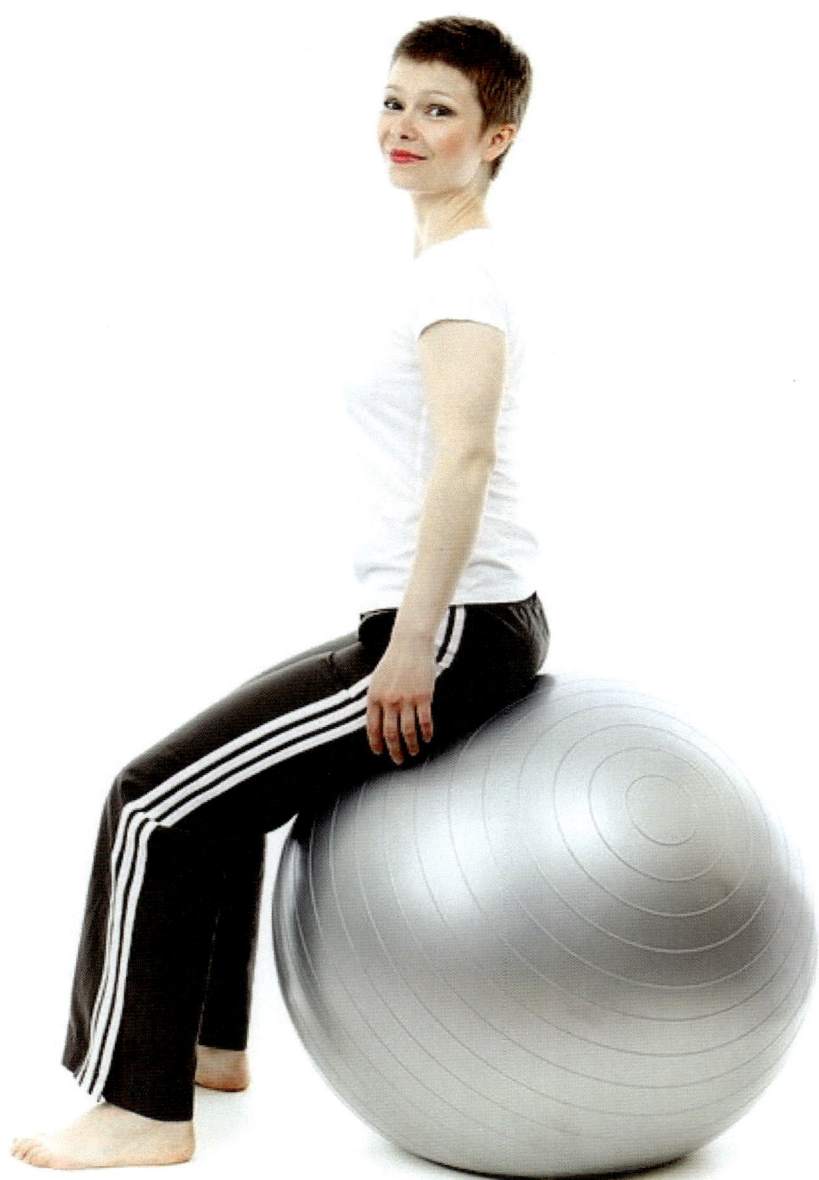

Another simple exercise you should try is to stand up straight next to a wall and have the ball between your rear end and the wall. Then you simply balance like this and perhaps lean carefully towards the wall back and forth. People with back problems often have a good experience from this exercise and it is a good change for your entire body if you are normally sitting still a lot.

A third exercise that is popular as well is when you start by sitting on the ball, then place your feet 12 inches apart on the floor. Next, stick your arms up and out in the air for balance. Raise one of your legs above the floor, about 1 inch up in the air. Try to keep your leg like this for 30 minutes. If it is too hard, just take it down and try again. When you are finished with one leg, take the other one and do the same thing. This exercise will of course also be easier to do after you have done it several times. Remember, these exercises are good if you repeat them often, in your normal exercise routine. If you would like to know more exercises using a fitness ball, just simply search for it on the internet, there are many!

Using a jumping rope
Jumping rope (or rope skipping) is one of the best ways to work on conditioning from your home. You can find jumping

ropes under 5 dollars (I recommend a lightweight plastic rope for beginners), and they are also easy to bring with you on vacations etc. 9-foot ropes are common, but do try the length in the store if possible. Most of us have tried jumping rope before, but few of us do it as adults in regular workout programs. That is shame, given that jumping rope improves ones coordination, endurance, quickness and footwork.

For those of you who don't know, you start with the rope on the floor behind your back, and then you swing it forwards over your head and you jump, almost simultaneously, so it swishes under your feet whilst your body is in the air. Then you repeat it without stopping. There are of course variations to jumping rope, but this is the common approach.

However, if you are not familiar with jumping rope, you will find that it is more difficult and testing than you might think. This exercise really needs practicing and repetition. So, my advice if you feel like getting started with the rope is that you start easily, for just 20-30 seconds in a row the first days, and then slowly try it for a little longer sequence and go from there. For athletes, it is common practice to jump rope in rounds with small pauses between them. Once you feel somewhat comfortable with jumping rope, try to make a suitable program of rounds, for example 4 x 2 minutes, with a 60 second break between the rounds.

It is hard jumping rope in the beginning as regards balance and coordination. It also takes a lot of energy, focus and space, so make sure to stand on a wide empty floor (a floor that is not too sensitive as this exercise might leave marks on the floor, depending on the fabric). There are appropriate carpets you can buy and use if you don't want to perform this exercise on your living room floor. If you have a garden or a backyard, then those are great place as well for jumping rope.

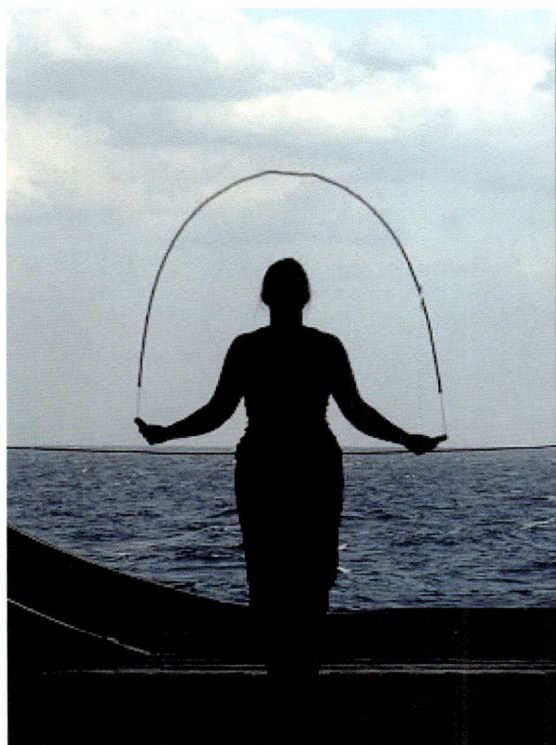

Chapter 7: Positive reinforcements for a much healthier you

While regular physical activity and a healthy diet play major roles in attaining and maintaining a fit and healthy body, it is also important to be aware of the very fact that our other actions and habits could also significantly affect the state of our health and our overall wellbeing.

In order to fully enjoy the benefits of exercising and healthy dieting, these healthy and positive reinforcements are also needed in order to truly become better and much healthier:

- *Drink an adequate amount of water daily.*

   Water is among our basic needs because of the very fact that without it, we would certainly perish. It is a vital element needed by our body to function at its best. The body utilizes water for the transport of nutrients throughout the body, for body temperature regulation, chemical and metabolic reactions, elimination of waste, and to sustain cell life.

   Not only does water perform these vital functions but they are also a good and healthy way to freshen up especially during warm days!

- *Manage stress.*

Aside from being an ultimately unpleasant experience, it is also important to be aware that stress also has a way of making your various body functions go all awry.

Stress hormones could affect your cardiovascular and respiratory systems and cause blood vessels to constrict and as a result, raise blood pressure. Chronic stress is also known to increase your risk of having a stroke or a heart attack and of developing certain health conditions, such as type 2 diabetes. Stress could also set off an unhealthy cycle by affecting your mood which in turn, could affect your motivation to exercise or follow a healthy diet.

While stress is a normal part of life, we must make an effort to be able to manage it well. It cannot be totally eliminated from our lives but what we can actually do is to find more productive ways on how to deal with them instead.

- *Always find time to rest.*

With our very busy lifestyle nowadays, we tend to overwork our body and we often forget that we also need to rest just as much as we need to be physically active. When we rest, we significantly give our body the opportunity it needs to renew, repair and recover from all the hard work done during the day. It also helps recharge our energy levels, allowing us to be fully functional when we are awake.

Preferably, we should be able to obtain eight hours of restful sleep each night. Inadequate rest and constant sleep deprivation could result to stress and lethargy, both of which could significantly affect our efforts of exercising and dieting.

If we lose our health, then we also lose the chance to experience life. Thus, for each new morning, we must take it as another wonderful opportunity to make healthy and positive changes in our lives.

The road towards becoming better and healthier does not have to entail drastic and difficult changes. It just has to be taken one little step at a time. Be mindful of your goal and be patient yet consistent with your tiny efforts. This is the very key that will open the way towards actually living a healthy, happy and better lifestyle.

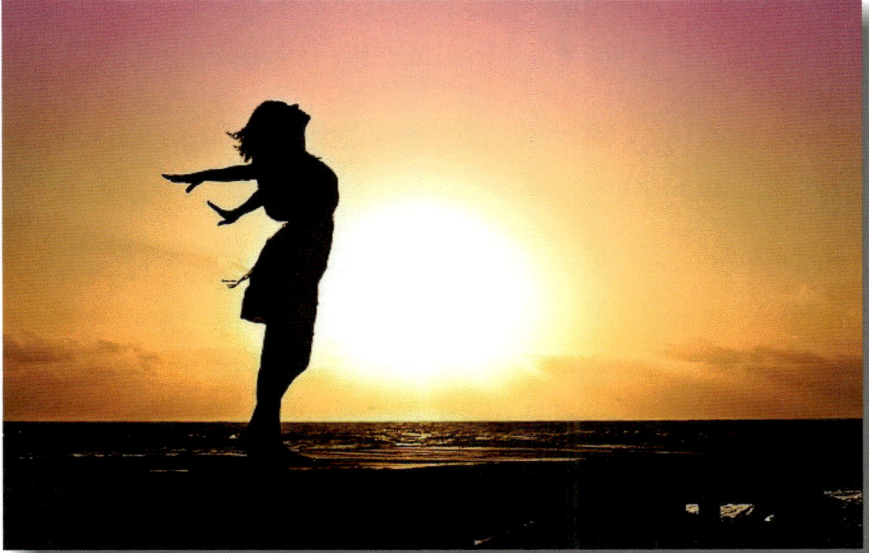

Conclusion

Thank you again for downloading this book!

I hope this book was inspirational and able to help you start working out at home.

With these workout exercises described above, you need to eat properly as well. A crappy diet and a good workout will take you nowhere. Eat fruits, nuts, and vegetables etc. Try eating natural, whole foods and quit drinking soda, eating junk and candy. Your diet can be a big part of your failure or success.

Now that you have hopefully made a plan for yourself with some of the exercises provided in this book, the next step is to follow it so that you will get the results that you want and deserve. Keep in mind that this plan should not be written in stone, feel free to adapt it and change it over time so that it fits your individual needs. Do not also forget to combine these exercises with walking or jogging regularly.

Motivation is an essential thing to have when beginning to workout. Enjoy the exercises you do and remember not to exhaust your body so much. Do as much your body can easily bear. When you begin, start with easy workouts. When your body is used to the easy workouts, only then should you start with intense workouts. Go slow! Do not rush things.

The more you enjoy doing these exercises, the more effective they will be. Finally, if you enjoyed this book, then I would like to ask you for a favor, would you be kind enough to leave a small review for this book on Amazon? It would be greatly appreciated!

Thank you and good luck with your workout!

Elle Petersen

If you liked reading this book, then I would also love for you to check out my other book *'Exercise and Fitness over 50',* which I believe might suit you as well. Enjoy a preview on the following pages and then check it out online if you would like to know more about the book.

Preview of 'Exercise and Fitness over 50'

Chapter 6: How to integrate exercises into your daily routine

While a single day of not being able to exercise would not likely have an immediate, unfavorable effect on your health, it is important to realize that years, months, or even weeks of having too little physical activity could already greatly distress not just your body and your physical health, but the overall quality of your life as a whole as well. This is the very reason why it is very important that we are able to consistently incorporate daily exercises into our daily lives.

However, for a lot of individuals, the thought of exercising every single day may seem a bit overwhelming or may even seem impossible especially for individuals who are bound to a tight schedule.

So how exactly will you add more movement and physical activity to your day to day routine even despite a very hectic schedule? Here are some practical tips and tricks on how to find more opportunities for exercising throughout the day:

→ Do your exercises first thing in the morning. Make it a point to get up twenty or thirty minutes earlier than usual and do your workouts before the day starts and before any other tasks distract you from doing so.

→ Stretching is considered to be a simple yet very great form of exercise and can even be done several times throughout the day with minimum effort. In between your various tasks during the day, try pausing for a few moments to take a short break and to simply stretch your limbs.

→ Seize every little opportunity to walk. Take the stairs instead of the escalator or elevator. Walk to work if possible (if you still work, that is). Pace around while talking to someone on the phone. Take a short walk if you need to ponder on something. Get up and walk towards the television to change channels instead of using the remote control. Take a walk around the house while waiting for the pot to boil. Again, take every single opportunity no matter how small.

→ During work breaks, spend a few minutes stretching, walking, or climbing stairs.

→ While watching television at home, jog in place, do leg exercises, or lift some weights during commercial breaks.

→ Perform some of the household chores manually. Water the plants, sweep or mop the floor manually, weed the garden, rake those autumn leaves, or shovel some snow. Make these house chores an opportunity to exercise and improve your health.

→ During vacations, make it a point to go outdoors to do something more physically active. And in order to make these activities both physically and emotionally rewarding, perform these activities with your loved ones. Clean the backyard together, head to the beach, go camping, play some sport, or simply take a walk towards the park together.

These simple physical activities may not be as dynamic as the kinds of exercises and workouts performed by individuals in the gym. But no matter how small these activities are, the benefits and the rewards that they could bring to your health and your overall wellbeing in the long run are surprisingly great and largely significant.

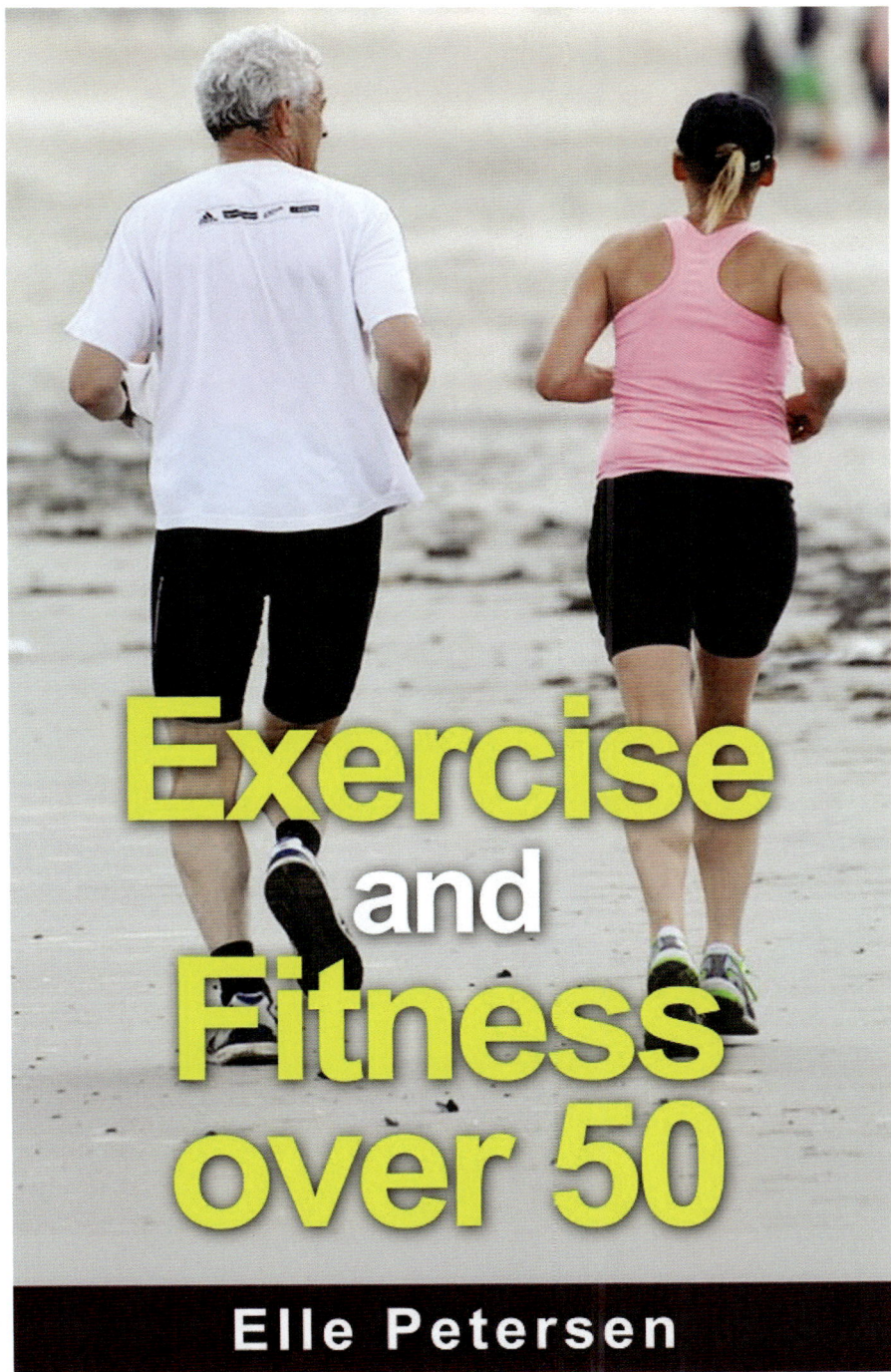

Exercise and Fitness over 50

Elle Petersen

Printed in Great Britain
by Amazon